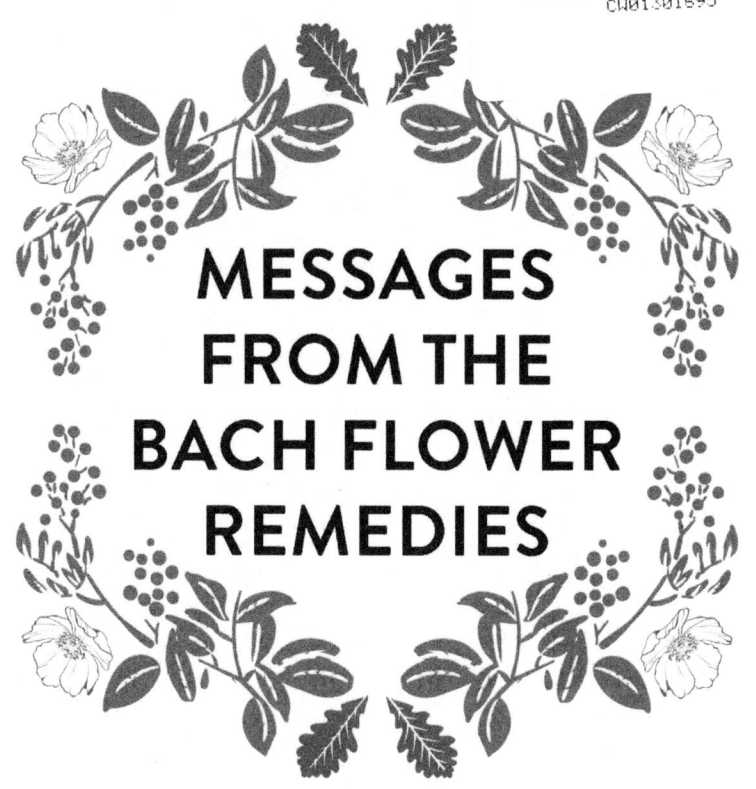

MESSAGES FROM THE BACH FLOWER REMEDIES

An Oracle Book

Written by Helen Scott

With love from me + the flowers!

Helen Scott

Copyright © 2023 Helen Scott

All rights reserved.

No part of this publication may be reproduced, stored in a retrieval system, or transmitted in any form or by any means, electronic, mechanical, photocopying, recording or otherwise, without the prior written permission from both the copyright owner and publisher.

CONTENTS

Introduction   1
Dr Edward Bach and the Bach Flower Remedies   3
How to Use This Book   6
Agrimony   8
Aspen   10
Beech   12
Centuary   14
Cerato   16
Cherry Plum   18
Chestnut Bud   20
Chicory   22
Clematis   24
Crab Apple   26
Elm   28
Gentain   30
Gorse   32
Heather   34
Holly   36
Honeysuckle   38
Hornbeam   40
Impatiens   42
Larch   44
Mimulus   46

Mustard	48
Oak	50
Olive	52
Pine	54
Red Chestnut	56
Rock Rose	58
Rock Water	60
Scleranthus	62
Star of Bethlehem	64
Sweet Chestnut	66
Vervain	68
Vine	70
Walnut	72
Water Violet	74
White Chestnut	76
Wild Oat	78
Wild Rose	80
Willow	82

*In memory and gratitude
of Uncle Alan*

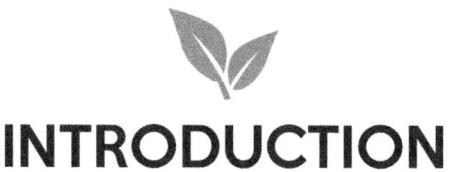

INTRODUCTION

This book can be used in many ways. It is an oracle, a book of wisdom, a perspective on the Bach flowers, an overview of the human characteristics and potentially the seed to much more. This book was created to give the Bach flowers a voice.

We discuss them usually in regard to symptoms versus balanced state; human observations to how the vibrations of the plant interact with our energy field and the changes they induce. This is indeed useful, and how Dr Bach created and introduced us to the remedies. If you are new to the Bach flower remedies, it might be useful to get one of the many books that describes them in this way as it provides you with a good overview.

It is not, however, necessary to have any knowledge of the Bach flower remedies to use this book. The wisdom contained within it is relevant to all humans with a personality. We all have these aspects, gifts and challenges on some level, some affecting us more than others. If you are knowledgeable in the Bach flowers, then this book can offer another level of understanding. A perspective from the plants themselves. A dialogue between the plant kingdom and humanity. A reflection on how two forms of consciousness, of vibration, of energy, can come together.

Each flower brings its own seed of wisdom to plant within you. These seeds will not suddenly turn into blooming flowers straight away; however, with patience, attention, and the right conditions, they will grow. Once fully in bloom you may become the embodiment of this wisdom yourself. Or maybe the seed will lay dormant for many years, until the right conditions arise, and suddenly it will sprout to life. Trust in the speed and patterns of nature, and you may find your life greatly enhanced.

This book was written in an urban area of Manchester, in the North of England. Not in some idyllic garden or place in nature, but surrounded by red brick terraced houses, inner city streets and very few plants. It was written by taking these essences and quietly listening. These essences can be a portal to nature, even when nature can be hard to find.

A powerful way to use this book is alongside the essences. To take a few drops, quieten down, read the plant's wisdom, then listen to your own personal message from within (if you can get quiet enough to hear it). How do the messages and the essences resonate within your being? What aspects of yourself are triggered and revealed? Watch as the medicine of the messages and vibrations of the plants softly and slowly unfurl you much like the petals of a rose basking in the sun.

DR EDWARD BACH AND THE BACH FLOWER REMEDIES

Dr Edward Bach was an English physician, bacteriologist and homeopath who lived from 1886 to 1936. Before moving into the field of complementary medicine, he worked in conventional medicine and was well respected, working from a highly successful practice in Harley Street, London. However, Bach became dissatisfied with the traditional approach of treating physical symptoms alone and moved towards a more holistic approach to healing. He understood that emotional and mental imbalances were at the root of many physical illnesses. This led him to explore a more natural, alternative approach to health and healing.

In the 1930s, Dr Bach identified 38 different remedies, each corresponding to a specific emotional state or personality trait. These remedies are made mostly from the flowers of certain plants and trees, which are infused in water to capture their vibrational properties. To create the remedies, Bach used a technique known as "the sun method". He would place the flowers in a bowl of pure water and set the bowl in direct sunlight for several hours. The sunlight would transfer the vibrational energy of the flowers to the water. Some of the remedies were made by "the boil method", which involved boiling the plants. The essence made—the mother essence—was further diluted and preserved with brandy to create the stock remedies, which can then be diluted further and combined with multiple remedies.

The Bach flower remedies help to address emotional issues including fear, anxiety, stress, and lack of confidence. They support the receiver into transforming these issues into a more positive state. They are a form of complementary medicine and are a support to emotional well-being rather than treating physical ailments directly.

To select the appropriate remedy, a person can consider their emotional state and choose a remedy that matches their issues, or even better, consult with a trained practitioner. This book can assist in supporting the reader to select the remedies needed. Each remedy is believed to address a specific emotional state and help restore balance. The remedies can be taken orally, either directly from the bottle or by diluting it further in water, and can also be applied topically or added to bath water. There are many creative ways to work with these essences you can discover if you wish to explore further.

Dr Bach's work and the flower remedies grew popular during his lifetime and continues to be used by people seeking a more holistic approach to emotional healing and well-being. The Bach flower remedies are still widely available today and used by many people worldwide. When using the Bach flower remedies, it's important to remember they are not a substitute for professional medical care, and consulting a healthcare advisor is recommended when considering physical ailments.

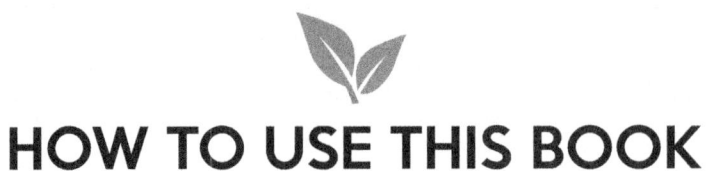

HOW TO USE THIS BOOK

AS AN ORACLE BOOK

Take a breath, and open the book at a random page. Which of the Bach flower remedies presents themselves to you and wishes to share their wisdom? Is it relevant to your past, your present, or possibly your future? Maybe the message will be received loud and clear, or maybe a seed of understanding is gently emerging. Invite yourself to meditate on the message and allow its wisdom to germinate.

AS A REMEDY COMPANION

This book can be read alongside taking the Bach flower remedies. Let the energy of the flowers within the essence you take work through your system, whilst regularly reading the message of the remedy within this book. Helping you to receive and embody the wisdom and message.

AS A REFERENCE

To study the Bach flower remedies, the human condition, and the rich experience of life.

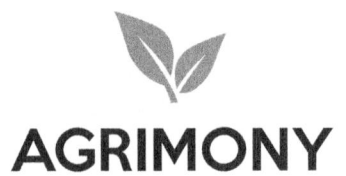

AGRIMONY

Symptoms: cheerful face hiding mental torture

Positive effects: inner peace, open, honest

I am here to show you the forgotten parts of life. The uncomfortable aspects of yourself which are suppressed and denied. We often wish to hide certain parts of ourselves from others. This is the same as society not wanting to recognise the vulnerable, so we hide them from view. Moving on the homeless, hiding away the ill, criminalising the addict does not solve the problem.

Within yourself I ask you to honour the vulnerable, give space for the damaged. A happy face and a saddened heart are a form of self-neglect. Like having a favourite child who displays all the traits you like and admire. You lavish this "child" with attention, showing them off to the world. The other child who may display not so savoury traits—selfishness, moodiness, shyness—you lock away, choosing to focus on the perfected image. The damage to the neglected child, rather than healing, brings on further damage.

Hidden away in a secret room, developing feelings of shame and unworthiness.

I ask that you would not do this to a child, so why treat yourself with such neglect? I can help support you in gently opening the doors of the rooms hiding those aspects of yourself that remain unloved and rejected.

Acknowledgement on its own can be incredibly healing. Before acknowledgement, no healing of these traits or the self as a whole is possible.

RESISTANCE TO HEALING - AGRIMONY

I ask you not to be scared of rejection from others. Until you stop rejecting yourself, rejection will always be a fear that has a hold on you. In order to move away from a fear of rejection, this self-acknowledgement is needed. There is no rush. You can open the door and peer round in your own time.

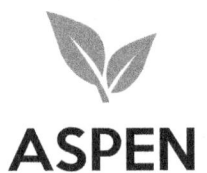

ASPEN

Symptoms: fear of unknown things

Positive effects: reassured, calm, trusting

I am here to show you the love buried beneath your fear. The excitable nature of your emotions gets distracted like a magpie searching for shiny things: reaching you for fearful feelings, unable to put them down. Like a magnet you attract dread and anxiety—you see it lurking in darkened corners. Unsure what is there to fear, this leads to further anticipation of doom.

But ... there is nothing there! Nothing to fear. But something draws you back. An unconscious connection to the mysterious frightening realms. A nightmare within waking life with no obvious plot or meaning.

I ask you to settle. Allow me to turn down the dial of this frequency you are tuned to. Beneath this fog of fear lies a still deep pool of love. It has always been there, waiting for you to discover.

See the fear settling like autumn leaves dropping from the tree and settling to the ground. The leaves shivering on the tree serve no purpose now. Distracting you from the solid truck of the tree, the roots reaching down ground you into the earth. Strong, rooted and still. Reaching down to the nurture below and stretching up towards love.

Allow me to gently wash away the fear. Let me lead you to the pool. Let me uncover your solid, rooted trunk that was there all the time. Let me help you rest in love.

RESISTANCE TO HEALING – ASPEN

What if I lose my fearful nature? Something terrible might happen! If I rest in love, I might get caught off guard! Emotions can be addictive. We believe we thrive and survive on that which is holding us back. The most powerful, protective state is love. I suggest you have tried fear, terror and anxiety and it has not been effective in providing security. Let me point you in the direction of soft, still love, and you can experience for yourself and make your choices from there.

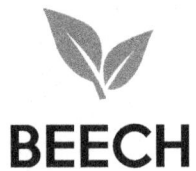

BEECH

Symptoms: intolerance, perfectionist

Positive effect: tolerance, understanding

I am here to teach you the wonder of tolerance. To walk through the world with ease and grace, surrounded by irritants and annoyances, but to glide straight through. Peacefully observing.

This is not denial of difficult situations or people. It is still possible to look directly at these disturbing scenarios, but not be entwined in the friction of clashing vibrations.

See yourself as covered in a grease, an oil, a divine lubrication. The minute friction comes into your life, unless you want to get stuck, slide through. Friction can cause irritation, intolerance. An emotional rise in judgement, anger, jealousy, disappointment … the list goes on. This can lead to an understanding of your own issues to heal, but it is much kinder to yourself to observe this from an objective place of peace. I am here to help you extinguish the friction, disturbance, and intolerance of your world. Rather than creating further disturbing resonances by adding emotions to fuel the fire.

Imagine you only had an itchy woollen jumper to wear. It was your only option and there was no escaping it. I am the energy of tolerance. A silk shirt between the rough, irritating jumper and your sensitive skin. The jumper is the same jumper, your experience is completely different.

Tolerance of the world is the path to peace. With eyes open to the difficulties and willingness to change things. Without being swept along with the emotional, judgemental storms.

RESISTANCE TO HEALING – BEECH

But I can see clearly all the wrongs around me, and I refuse to deny them! You may say this in all righteousness. And you may have a point! Can you change things? Yes—then change them. Can you speak up? Then speak up. What can you do? If there is nothing you can do, then you are only fighting yourself with a tornado of intolerant emotions. Until you let go and allow these feelings to slide away to a place of tolerance and acceptance, you will never find peace.

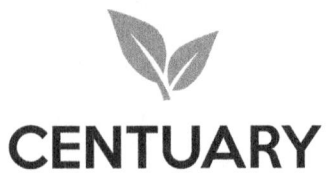

CENTUARY

Symptoms: difficulty saying no, submissive

Positive effects: assertive, strength

I am here to teach you of your significance and importance. There is no pecking order in the divine order of things. This is created by personalities placing themselves where they think they deserve to be. You are equal. You are important. You deserve to have your needs met.

A perfect example of this is in an emergency on an airplane and the oxygen masks falls. You are asked to put your own on before you help anyone else, including children and the vulnerable. This is because you are no use to anyone if you do not help yourself first.

You are number one in your own life. This is not selfish. This is common sense. How can you achieve all you want and live the life you were meant to if your needs are bottom of the pile? Also, are there some selfish motives to needing to be needed? Is that where you find your self-worth, or try to? By becoming indispensable in other people's lives so you might have a chance of becoming important? But instead, you become taken for granted and used with an expectation that you will always be there. A doormat.

Find your importance within yourself! We are all worthy and deserving of love and respect, but this must come from within us for us to truly experience it.

RESISTANCE TO HEALING -CENTUARY

People will not manage without me! They need me! If I put myself first, I am denying someone else!

This is a self-imposed prison, for yourself and possibly for the others you think you are helping. You are interrupting the flow of lessons and learnings and personal responsibility. The world will go on without you. Is that a thought that fills you with fear, or liberation?

By elevating yourself to a place of self-respect and equal importance, not only do you set yourself free, but also the others you love.

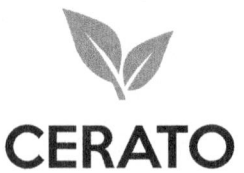

CERATO

Symptoms: indecision and self-doubt

Positive Effects: intuition, self-belief

I am here to teach you that your own mind and heart are the most valuable assets you have. It is only when you look within for the answers do you truly find the truth and direction you desire. Why then, do you cast out your wisdom and replace it with the second-rate opinions of others? No one else can compare to your inner voice yet you are continually grasping for guidance outside of yourself. Pestering and pecking the minds of others. By doing this you are diverting responsibility. Attempting to make others responsible for your actions, decisions, and mistakes. Then you can lay blame outside of yourself when things do not go to plan.

Become quiet. Learn to seek silence first. Practice going within. For underneath all the questions you so desperately wish to be answered, are the answers. Find the stillness and you won't even have to ask the questions. You will know when you need to know.

We all have the inner resources, we just need to be guided towards them. Others can be signposts, pointing us in the right direction; however, they can also lead you down the wrong path.

You have within you all you need to know. Keep quieting, looking within, until you find that voice, that space, that void, which tells you all you need to know when you need to know it.

RESISTANCE TO HEALING – CERATO

But I do not know what to do! I have people all around me who are so wise! I would be foolish not to take their advice! Trust yourself. Get to know yourself. Find your wisdom. Make mistakes. You may not always have wise people around, and truly wise people would encourage you to find your own answers.

Many fools masquerade as wisdom keepers, to feed their insecurities. How can you possibly think anyone else's options are better than you own inner wisdom?

Until you take responsibility for yourself, owning your victories and failures, you will never be fully at ease.

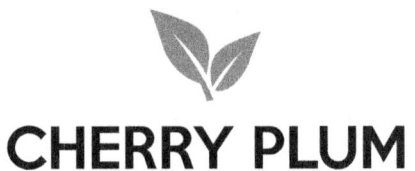

CHERRY PLUM

Symptoms: fear of losing control

Positive effects: composure, security, self-control

I am here to teach you strength and resilience. You can sometimes be at the point of breaking. Your hands grasping onto the window ledge, forgetting who you are or where your senses have gone. You have lost control and your legs are scrambling beneath you, trying to find solid ground where there is none.

The world can be an overwhelming place. The pressures and strains can be so much it is tempting to lose ourselves in a madness, a breakdown, a violent place of destruction and debilitation.

Why did you find yourself on that ledge when it all got too much? Have you not just made your predicament worse? Would it not have been easier to survey this overwhelming situation or feeling from the safety of looking out of the window? The problems may still be there, but you are stoic and steadily surveying them. What use are you as a raging out of control flame, trying to burn away your existence?

As you move into a state of disassociation you only delay the inevitable reality, often adding further consequences. I am here to teach you strength and resilience are the key when overwhelmed. The minute you try to run away from yourself, stop. Take a breath, take another breath. You are still here. You can deal with this. You will recover.

RESISTANCE TO HEALING – CHERRY PLUM

But I just cannot cope! Is adding extreme distress a better solution? Is complete loss of control going to help? Finding acceptance of the moment you are in, knowing you can only deal with one moment at a time, will gradually lead you to the strength and resilience you need to get back to life equilibrium. No matter your outer circumstances.

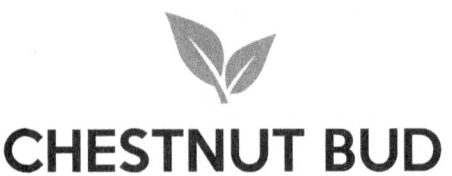

CHESTNUT BUD

Symptoms: failure to learn from mistakes

Positive effects: insight, observant, reflective

I am here to show you the true value of your life experiences. You find yourself stumbling through life having the same set of circumstances repeating themselves over and over. Your life is a broken record. You feel like a victim—*why does this always happen to me?*

You are stuck on the same level, like a computer game. It is getting boring, uncomfortable and frustrating. How do you complete this part of the game? You look for clues. You pay attention. You try a different method. You reflect on how you could have done things differently.

If you are finding things in your life repeating in ways you do not wish, then the only way out is to look at your part in the picture. What is life trying to teach you? What are you missing? Reflect and then respond and you can make it to the next level, the next experience, which will more than likely be a positive change.

We see you rushing around walking into the same lamppost over and over. Take note. Notice what is in front of you and learn to avoid the hazards set in your way. But these hazards are valuable. They are doorways to new opportunities if used correctly. But they are also holes you can fall into, sending you back to repeat the cycle until you finally learn.

RESISTANCE TO HEALING – CHESTNUT BUD

Your life is calling for change, but you resist. It might not be perfect, but this is what you know and what has become your accepted reality. Do you not deserve more? Do you not want to hear that next song on the record? If you are truly stuck in life and in acceptance of this, you are not truly living.

Only when you open your eyes and be responsible for the actions you take will you be able to transcend this monotonous recurring dream.

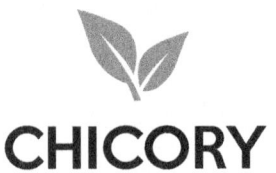

CHICORY

Symptoms: possessive love, clingy, smothering

Positive effects: unconditional love, selfless

I am here to teach you to trust in the process of life. Why focus so much on the lives of others? How will your expectations of what is best for them ever compare to the wisdom of their own journey? And how is their journey comparable to your own?

I am here to highlight that your own path is the one you should be giving your attention. By involving yourself in others, you find yourself walking on their path, putting 'helpful' obstacles in their way, possibly diverting them from the important mistakes and lessons that their soul so wishes them to partake in. Meanwhile, your path is neglected. Weeds grow on your soul's precious route as it is not being trod. The result of which, those around you have paths that seem ever more attractive to you.

STOP. Take a look around. Where is your attention? Is it outside yourself.? Desperately trying to manipulate life into a controllable picture of happiness? The result of which can have the opposite effect of your desire. Pushing loved ones away as they try and reclaim a path of their own. Your path once loved is beautiful. Reclaim it and allow those around you to rejoice in its splendour. You are unique, as are those around you, and you are loved just as you are.

RESISTANCE TO HEALING – CHICORY

But if I let go of others, I might lose them! If you hold on too tightly you are more likely to lose them. You grip on worrying you might lose control of your outside world. You are putting your power outside of yourself. By turning inwards, focusing on your inner world, you can begin to feel the security and love you so much want in your life.

Let go of your outer world and focus on the inner. Become receptive to your true path.

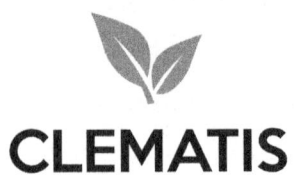

CLEMATIS

Symptoms: dreaming of future, inattentive, absentminded

Positive effects: focus, grounded, action, clear

I am here to teach you the value of being present in your circumstance. It is where you are ALWAYS meant to be. Here, now. Not in some perfected distant future, not floating high in some deluded fairy tale. Here. Now.

Your desire to escape life only prolongs the pain. Your escapist attempts might feel good in the moment, but they resolve nothing that needs resolving. Would it not be better to experience what your soul so wishes for you to experience, rather than some fantastical creation that is some makeshift coverup to hide your pain? Life can be painful. But you can cope with it. Unless it is found hidden in the back of that old cupboard, long forgotten and brought into the light to be witnessed, it will always be there. And you will always be avoiding, ignoring and pretending what is in front of you isn't there.

Imagination can be a wonderful thing. An extremely useful tool to create infinite positive possibilities. It can also be a destructive distraction.

Feel your body walking on the earth. Notice where you are. If you do not like what you feel, is there something you can do to change how you feel? If you ignore it and spend your life floating about not registering what is in front of you it is impossible to feel fulfilled. Fulfilment is where your soul is fully present, filling your body with its full attention. Living the life it has come to live.

RESISTANCE TO HEALING – CLEMATIS

But I do not want to be here! I did not choose this life! But you are, and you did. There is no escape. Your pain does not disappear unless you address it. Stop sugar coating and avoiding. You are only creating yourself more pain and suffering.

Be gentle and begin with small steps. Step out into nature. Take in the sights, smells and sensations. Is it not beautiful? Could your life not be this beautiful? Maybe it already is but you're too busy avoiding it to give a moment's notice to appreciate the beauty of where you already are.

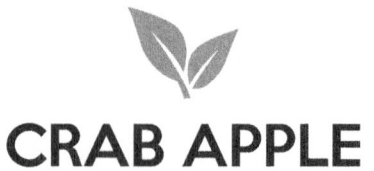

CRAB APPLE

Symptoms: cleansing, self-loathing, impurity

Positive effects: self-love, self-acceptance, purity

I am here to teach you about the purity of life. You see imperfections, dirt, infections, and disease all around. But what about the oyster that turns a piece of grit into a pearl? These are the materials needed to turn lead into gold. Alchemy of the soul. Without these imperfections there would be no life, no challenge, no drive for transformation. But instead, you feel trapped by illness, by the drudge, by the dirt. Weighed down by your darkness and that of the world around you, you feel an obsessive need to focus on what is wrong, what is there to hinder you, why you are stuck in place of squalor and misery.

But our planet is made out of dirt, bacteria is needed, emotions are necessary. Embrace this world. Accept it for what it is and anything holding you back, recognise it is possible to transform. If not on the outside, then on the inside.

Purity is a state of seeing everything just as it is. Detached, yet connected. All in perfect balance. Constantly changing, rebalancing. See yourself as part of this constant change, like nature. Growth and decay—both of equal importance. Without one we cannot have the other.

RESISTANCE TO HEALING – CRAB APPLE

But I need to keep on top of the dangers, there is contamination all around! Why are you judging what is good and what is bad? Is it not all just a part of your experience? Is your outer circumstance and surroundings not just a perfect mirror to as how you perceive the world?

With a change of perception, you can see with different eyes. The world is set up to support you and your own personal perception. To find purity in your life, you must find purity within.

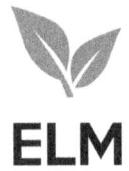

ELM

Symptoms: overwhelmed by responsibility

Positive effects: capable, support, inner-reliability

I am here to teach you that no matter what life throws at you, you will always come through the other side of it. When life throws up what seems like too many responsibilities there is always the present moment to rest in. Life ebbs and flows, and when the flow seems too strong then stop. Rest in the present moment. Things will not fall to pieces if you take some time to rest.

Have you taken on too much? Can you prioritise, delegate, or drop certain responsibilities you have taken on? Is it possible to ask for help? You do not need to carry the weight of the world on your shoulders. If all the things in your life do need you to carry them, trust that you will never be given more than you can handle. Trust that even if things seem to go wrong and it all becomes too much, this is not a failure. This is another opportunity for growth. Trust in the process. Trust that there will be moments of calm along the way. Trust you are good enough, whatever the outcome.

And do not forget the present moment, and opportunity to let things go. Just five minutes and you can rest in the stillness. Let everything fall away. Things will not fall apart if you take a break. Allow yourself space to release the inner feelings of overwhelm, then return to the task at hand, clearer, calmer. You can only do one thing at a time. And when the panic rises and it all seems too much, remind yourself once more that the present moment is always here and now to rest in.

RESISTANCE TO HEALING – ELM

But if I stop thinking about everything at once it may all fall to pieces! If you try to think of everything all at once, then you will fall to pieces! Allow the efficiency and organisation of the present moment to flood your being. Notice how, in the stillness, things seem to fall into place. Trying to control everything in your mind only leads to mental exhaustion and overwhelm. This time will pass. You are enough.

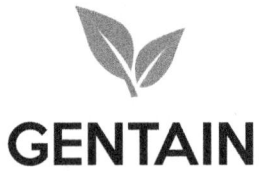

GENTAIN

Symptoms: discouragement after a setback, pessimism, doubt

Positive effects: optimism, encouragement

I am here to teach you the value of rising above the self-imposed negative outlook. Why the doom and gloom? What purpose is it showing you? How is it possibly helping you? If nothing seems to be going your way, have you asked yourself why?

A pessimistic outlook is as unrealistic as an optimistic one. They are both imaginings of fantasy outcomes. Instead, would it not be better to see and feel things as they are? See them without this self-inflicted filter of life being against you. And once this haze lifts you are able to let the light shine on glimmers of hope. These glimmers of hope are signposts to a more positive path. A life worth living. Would you not rather seek a life worth living than slowly grind to a halt and give up?

Open your eyes to what is in front of you. Begin with gratitude for the small things. The bright colour of a beautiful flower, the breeze against your skin. Allow this light to permeate your experience. Then notice yourself. What are you grateful for within you? Start small. The ability to smell, the ability to digest food. These small moments of gratitude create chinks in your armour that allow the light of hope in. Keep practising gratitude, moving onto bigger things—you will find the light of hope is contagious.

RESISTANCE TO HEALING – GENTAIN

But all I see is doom and gloom. I am just telling it like it is! You create doom and gloom so well in your existence, do you think you may be equally successful creating hope and light?

Your experience reflects what you choose to focus on. Would you rather experience light or gloom? It truly is up to you. And while this shift in perspective may not happen instantly, practising gratitude for the small things starts you heading in the right direction. There is a better way, and you can find it.

GORSE

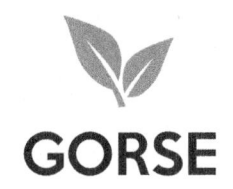

Symptoms: hopeless, despair, disheartened

Positive effects: renewed faith, hope

I am here to teach you that by entering the darkness, the gloom, hope is not lost. You may sit in these periods of despair to the point where they feel so familiar, you almost cannot remember how it felt to see the light, to feel uplifted.

But there is a point to these places. Once you are within them you can shine a light on what magnetises you to these pits of despair. Are you afraid of failure? Of not being enough? The world feels too heavy? By going to these dark places, you go to the roots of your unconscious fears. But these are fears. Not realities. There is no hope within these fears. But there is hope within yourself and, in fact, all around you. But it is hard to uplift yourself when the fears are calling you, hypnotising you. I ask you to sit in this place of gloom with new eyes, a new perspective. Are these fears really serving you? What is their purpose? Bring compassion into these gloomy thoughts, these unfounded fears. Do not reject them; embrace them as part of you. An expression of yourself that wanted to be found and noticed. But this expression of yourself can be changed with attention. Changed to a more useful thought. Feelings of hope and transformation CAN follow, and gratitude towards yourself for exploring the deep, dark caves within.

RESISTANCE TO HEALING – GORSE

But I cannot! I try—but it is all too heavy! It is all too much! Then do not try to escape it! Sit with your feelings gently and honestly. Have patience and compassion with yourself. Ask questions. *Why am I here?* You might find inner wisdom and insights by asking these questions. Or equally, you might hear the doom and gloom of your deepest subconscious. *Because I deserve to be. Because I fail in life. Because my life is hopeless.* Examine these statements. They want to be heard, examined, changed, and reframed. This is true healing.

HEATHER

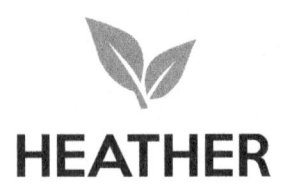

Symptoms: self-centred, self-concerned, talkative and lonely

Positive effects: empathy, good listener, comforted

I am here to teach you to be quiet. Stop a moment. Step back. You are grasping outside yourself for all your needs. Support, company, sympathy, acknowledgement. You are asking a lot of others, expecting them to fill you up, to work around you and to fulfil what you believe to be missing.

You are swallowing up the silence, the space, and the energies around you, like a big vacuum cleaner. But it is never enough!

Stop! Be quiet! Be still! Notice your surroundings! Open your eyes. The void you have been trying to fill is maybe what you have been craving all along. Maybe the healing you have being trying to find by filling up the space, filling up the emptiness, comes from the very places you have been trying to avoid.

Quiet. Peace. Solitude. These are essential experiences to master if you want to feel fully connected to others, your life, and your surroundings. Then you can achieve the fulfilling relationship with yourself and others you so deeply crave. There are more than likely other barriers within you to overcome before you can achieve this, but until you learn to be quiet you will force these potential paths to fulfilment firmly shut as you create every distraction possible.

RESISTANCE TO HEALING – HEATHER

But if we stop the conversation, stop the story, stop the experience, who will I be? What will I become? Where is my place? What is the worst that can happen? You are left with yourself in the emptiness. Well, maybe that is actually the best thing that can happen.

Has your technique worked yet? Has filling up the space led to fulfilment? I think not. You have got it all topsy turvy. Find the emptiness within the space to find true fulfilment. This may take time, but the time is now to take the U-turns and face the other way.

HOLLY

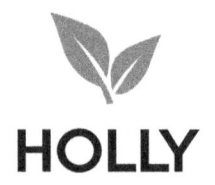

Symptoms: anger, hatred, envy, jealousy

Positive effects: love, acceptance, forgiveness

I am here to teach you the lesson of love and compassion. There are many injustices in our world. Many hurts, betrayals, abuses and the like. Sometimes bad things happen to good people. Sometimes good things happen to people who have lied and cheated their way to the top. Many reasons to be angry. Many reasons to cause jealousy.

This anger can maybe be justified in a desire for justice, a desire for change and equality. A call for action. If the changes can be made then this anger or envy can be the catalyst needed to put the change into action, which can move us into a place of love and peace. But what if this change cannot happen? Then we are left with anger, which can move into bitter hatred. Wishing for revenge or bad fortune for our enemies. A complete absence of love. And what does this achieve for ourselves? A cocktail of emotions that engulf us, clouding our perceptions to make the world and ugly, hateful place. We may have been justified in our anger originally, but if it festers within, all we are doing is poisoning ourselves.

The remedy is love. Loving our enemies. This is not condoning our enemy's behaviour. It is not settling for abuse and injustice. We can still see clearly what is unjust. We can just love whilst looking. This is true compassion. To be in every circumstance with love in our heart. Not contributing to the problem with hate but easing it with love.

RESISTANCE TO HEALING – HOLLY

But I hate it and I am so angry! I cannot let this go. Maybe you can't let it go, but maybe you can be connected in a state of love and compassion rather than anger and hatred. Easier said than done, but it is truly the only answer that can contribute to the solution in a positive way. You will only hurt yourself, and possibly others, if you operate from anger, jealousy and hate.

HONEYSUCKLE

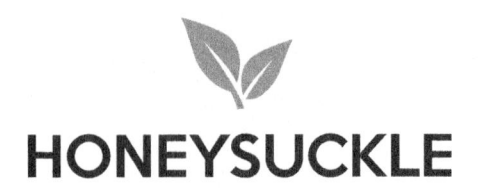

Symptoms: living in the past, overwhelming nostalgia

Positive effects: being present, letting go of the past

I am here to teach you the value of the present. To have your complete energy and attention anchored in the present moment is a powerful and beautiful experience. Even if your circumstances are not favourable at the present moment, it is still a perfectly profound experience to be fully present in the here and now.

The difficulty comes when your attention is taken away from the present moment. Back to some 'golden era' of the past. Or perhaps some haunting memory of a past regret. You begin to obsess, to over reflect on a mythical time within your own history. It is healthy to reflect on past experiences, but not to live in them. By dreamily reflecting you remove your energy from the true reality, your only real life—the present. The more you hark back to the past, the more your own lifeforce abandons you to live amongst the historic echoes of what you imagine to be your past.

You become a ghost of your former self, as you place most of your energy with your former self. Within this state the present is not a worthwhile place to be as your energy isn't present enough to experience what is under your nose.

It is time to call your soul back. Find out what you are missing now; do not regret missing it years down the line. What you see in front of you might surprise you.

RESISTANCE TO HEALING – HONEYSUCKLE

But I cannot let go of the past! It was just too important! Maybe it was THEN. But it is never as important as NOW. Reclaim the joy you imagine you felt in the past for NOW. Learn from the regrets you imagine from the past and bring that wisdom into the present. You are like a ghost who does not realise it's time to move on. A great future awaits you and it begins NOW!

HORNBEAM

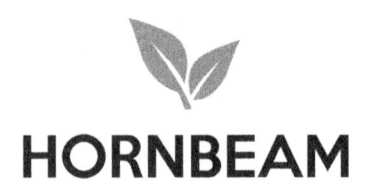

Symptoms: mental fatigue, procrastination

Positive effects: clarity, revitalised, resolve

I am here to teach you how to take things easy. To ease into things. To rest into the trust that things that need to be done, will be done.

When you have a mountain to climb, why waste your energy on fretting about how you will climb the mountain. Is it even possible? Will you have the energy? You will be exhausted before your first step. You will feel defeated before you have even tried. You have placed a range of mountains in front of the one you need to climb. No wonder you feel tired! But this energy is all wasted. Unnecessary effort expended in the imaginings of the mind. Make practical preparations—yes. But why waste your vital energy getting tired thinking about getting tired when there are real jobs to be done.

Rest in the energy of ease. Trust that you will be supported on your journey. It might be difficult, but you can do it! You are capable of the challenge. Cultivate the positive energy that will set the wind behind you on your journey, aiding your way up the mountain, rather than pacing around in circles in your mind, tiring yourself out and weighing you down. Would you not rather take the easy route? Let go of your self-made exhaustion. Believe in your path, believe in your role within upcoming challenges. There will be time to rest.

RESISTANCE TO HEALING – HORNBEAM

But it is all too much! What is all too much? Is it the actual work ahead, or is it your thoughts? Thinking takes up energy and you are overthinking. You can cope with what you are given. Trust yourself. And if you are right and it is too much then you can consider your options. But how do you know if you don't try? You might surprise yourself. But it will be easier with your batteries fully charged and not drained by your fears and mental exhaustion.

IMPATIENS

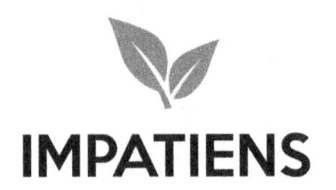

Symptoms: impatience, irritability, frustration

Positive effects: patience, ease tolerance

I am here to teach you patience. To trust in the flow of timings of all things. To find your own natural rhythms and to trust in the timings of others.

You are letting your mind run away with thinking it knows best. You are relying on what you think is correct speed, correct timing, rather than trusting in the perfection of divine timing. So, do you think you can do better than the forces of nature? Would you force a rose to open faster than its natural blooming? If so, you would damage or destroy it. The world would be less beautiful.

Can you not see the tasks and projects that need doing the same way? People have different rates of development, growing, blooming. Just like nature. Is a flower any better because it is quicker to grow and blossom? No. The same can be said for all things. Including people.

Patience in divine timing is the most efficient way to work. If you tap into this natural energy, you will understand that so much of your rushing is wasted energy. Sit back and wait until you know it is time. If setbacks happen, trust they are part of the process. If people are slow, communicate and assist if you need to. But ask yourself if you truly need to or is your mind and will taking over?

When you practice patience, things will fall into place almost like magic, and your life and those around you will benefit.

RESISTANCE TO HEALING – IMPATIENS

But people are not quick enough. If I do not do it, it just won't get done in time! Whose time? Are you setting yourself and others a speed that is out of touch with nature? Are you forgetting to stop and smell the roses? You may have forgotten that the collective journey is often more important than the destination. You rush things through losing touch with your surroundings. There is support all around you, but you miss out as you perceive it as not quick enough. Try the way of patience and discover the energy of grace.

LARCH

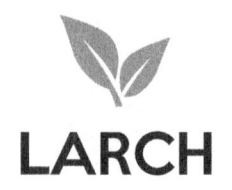

Symptoms: lack of confidence, fear of failure

Positive effects: self-confidence, self-esteem

I am here to teach you how valuable you are. How you are just as important and necessary as everyone else. How your role on this earth is a gift both to yourself and others.

You look around yourself, see other's successes and give up on yourself. Why bother even trying? You can never do anything good. Really? Think of all the things you have learnt to do well. Whether it is walking, talking, being kind, using a knife and fork. These are all miraculous achievements. And not everyone can do these things! Celebrate yourself. You are unique and talented in your own beautiful way.

Some people's role in life is grand and they seemingly achieve a lot. But along the way they might miss out on good relationships, noticing the world around them, communicating well. We all have a different role to play. Just because yours is different to those you see around you doesn't mean you should be disheartened.

Find out what brings your heart to life. What makes you feel joy when you think about it? It may be big, it may be small, but you have the freedom and capacity to get involved, whether it is a career or a hobby. You might not make big waves, but even small ripples make a difference to the world. Celebrate yourself and the person you came here to be!

RESISTANCE TO HEALING – LARCH

But there is not much point! Nothing I do will be worthwhile and someone could probably do it better than me. No one else can be you better than you! Stop with the comparisons and focus on what brings you joy. Is there a better achievement than bringing joy to the world? Your lack of confidence in the world could be limiting the joy in your life and therefore the amount of joy on the planet. Joy does not care about how well it's done. It is all about how much it is enjoyed. You cannot go wrong in joy.

MIMULUS

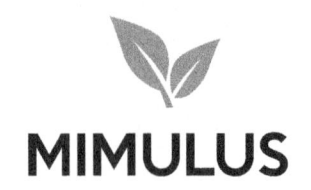

Symptoms: fear of known things, phobias, shyness

Positive effects: courage, security, safety

I am here to teach you strength. Strength of courage, strength of heart, strength of trust. There are many frightening things in the world and fear serves its purpose. It provides us with the fight or flight instincts which help us to survive. To continue living. But in our world, it is actually rare that this is needed. Yet we still live in fear. Fear of strangers, fear of open spaces, fear of spiders—the list goes on.

So, what purpose does fear serve other than to alert us to true danger? Rather than ensuring our survival, allowing us to keep living, it starts to do the opposite of its positive purpose. It stops us truly living. With fear coursing through our veins and systems, we become afraid of our own shadow. Jumpy, nervous and timid. The fear slowly weakens us, drains us of our strength. Our courage to face the world is even more diminished.

What if we could let the unnecessary fear go? What if all that energy used to fear what might happen, what you might experience or suffer, could go into truly living your life? Imagine the new source of strength you'd have. The courage to trust yourself, in the moment, if a dangerous or frightening experience ever occurred.

It is time to let go of fear. It does not serve you. You are strong and you are courageous. Your energies have just been temporarily distracted by fearful tales you have been telling yourself.

RESISTANCE TO HEALING – MIMULUS

But if I let my guard down, then something terrible will happen! How will I protect myself if I am not ready to react to these frightening things I am aware of? If something did happen to scare you, even something very frightening or traumatic, would you not be better equipped to deal with it from a place of strength, courage and trust, rather than a weakened, trembling state? You think you are preparing for the worst, but actually you are doing the opposite. You are living in the world from a fearful place therefore not fully living. You are not present to have all your energy ready to deal with whatever life throws your way.

MUSTARD

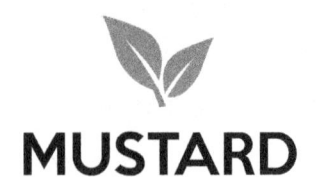

Symptoms: deep gloom for no reason, sudden melancholy

Positive effects: joy, brightness, clarity

I am here to teach you that even though dark, gloomy clouds may fill the sky, the sun is still behind them. All of a sudden, out of the blue, clouds may form covering the land below with darkness. This change of mood can be sudden and overwhelming. The sun, however, is still there. Much like a gloomy cloud casting shadows over your emotional mood. The darkness can almost fully black out the sun. But remember, it is still there.

And just as suddenly as the clouds appear, they can lift. Focus on the sun behind the clouds. Even if the gloom takes time to lift and there seems to be no reason for it hanging around, see it as a dark cloud covering the sun. The sun is just obscured. It is still there. The sun is permanent. The clouds are temporary. Just like our spirit and emotional state. Our spirit is like the sun. It is always there. It cannot be broken, just obscured. Our emotional state is temporary. It never stays the same. It can sometimes persist for a while, but a change in atmospheric conditions will always move it into a new state. Sometimes better, sometimes worse.

So, change the conditions! Go outside, take a walk, see a movie. Do anything to positively change the atmosphere. Eventually the gloomy clouds will lift to reveal your shining spirit that never left you. Your spirit is always with you, no matter how hidden.

RESISTANCE TO HEALING – MUSTARD

But I am too gloomy and low to see a movie! I cannot face taking a walk! Then start small. Set yourself a very small task. Tidy a small area of a room, draw a simple picture, do something slightly different, have tea instead of coffee. By doing something even just a little bit different it puts out the message that the atmosphere is changing. If you cannot face something, start smaller and build up. By changing the atmosphere in a positive way, no matter how small, the conditions for the clouds passing quickly become more favourable.

OAK

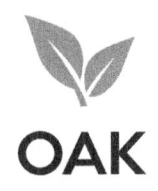

Symptoms: keeps going past point of exhaustion

Positive effects: strength, endurance, recharged

I am here to teach you of a most efficient power source you may have been overlooking. You may believe you have all the strength in the world. Making things happen, supporting your family, flying in your career. You push on and on, seeking success in all you do. Your efforts may pay off with achievements and accolades. But at what cost? Have you forgotten how to have fun? Have you forgotten how to play? This is understandable when you put all your energy into making things work for yourself and others. No time to rest, no time to relax. And if you delegate? The fear it will not get done to your high standards prevents you from asking for help.

So, you keep on pushing on and on. You have the energy. You can do it! You can achieve! Stop. As humans your energy is not unlimited. You have needs. To push on through, eats into your battery reserves. You are headed for burnout. Physically, mentally and emotionally.

But even when the signs are there you keep pushing through until you hit complete exhaustion and you have nothing left to give.

There is another way. Connect to a higher energy. Once tapped into this unlimited source you will understand the balance and timing of things. When to act, when to rest, when to play, when to retreat, when to connect, when to ask for help. You are supported by a spiritual energy. By continually pushing through you override the power of this energy and the support it brings. By tuning in the balance will come, things will get done, and life will become more joyful.

RESISTANCE TO HEALING – OAK

But I can do it! Watch me achieve! Watch me make things happen! Your strength can be immense, like a machine, efficiently powering through, getting the job done well. But machines break and then everything stops. They need to be well maintained, every aspect, every part looked after, or they will cease to function.

Your needs as a human need to be maintained or you will break. Find your true flow, let your will soften and allow balance to maintain you.

OLIVE

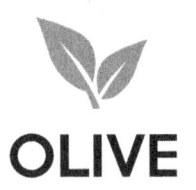

Symptoms: exhaustion

Positive effects: rejuvenation, vitality

I am here to teach you to rise out of exhaustion. Life can be exhausting. Illness, stress, life events can wear you down until the very act of existing can be too tiring. Everything is too much effort. I am here to reach my branch down into the hole that is so difficult for you to climb out of.

Take things slowly. If you are tired, then rest. Regain your strength. Be selective where you are using your energy and you will find your recovery back to health and vigour more rapid. If your health condition does not recover then by selectively using your energy you will regain inner strength, having more energy to get you through the day.

Energy sometimes needs to be rationed, to be prioritised. Finding ways you are burning your precious resources unnecessarily can be the key. Stress, worry, overthinking burns up fuel. If there is nothing you can do stop throwing logs onto that fire. Can some chores wait? When you are exhausted your priority is *you*. What can be put on the backburner until you have more fuel to spare?

Respecting your energy is the quickest route to recovery. The world keeps on spinning if you put off tidying up. When you have more energy, you can do it. Worrying about a messy room burns your precious resources. Wait until you have a well-stocked log pile until you can be more generous with your energy. With a bit of patience your body and mind will rebuild

RESISTANCE TO HEALING – OLIVE

But I am just so tired! I cannot seem to do anything! Then rest. Allow this vital time of recovery to rebuild. The stress of your exhaustion only leads onto further exhaustion. By accepting your situation and giving yourself the space to recover you conserve vital fuel. It is OK to rest. Charge your batteries. It is OK. Take your time. Rebuild your reserves. Look after yourself. It is OK to rest.

PINE

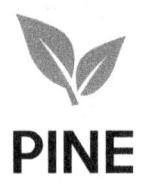

Symptoms: guilt, self-blame

Positive effects: freedom, self-forgiveness

I am here to teach you to trust yourself. You walk through life with guilt, seeing all the wrongs surrounding you and seeing your part in them, that you are responsible for. Even if a situation has nothing to do with you, you take a responsibility for it, apologetic and guilty. This leads to continuously berating yourself, beating yourself up just for being in the world.

Maybe you have made a mistake. Mistakes are part of being human. They are natural and can be healthy if we learn from them. They become unhealthy if we use them as a weapon against ourselves to inwardly torture, regret and blame.

You are no use imprisoned in guilt. You are not solving the situation you feel so bad about. It is time to trust yourself and your capacity to forgive and learn. Your capacity to let things go. Holding onto guilt is like a restraint, paralysing you so the only place for your mind to go is a spiral of mental self-harm.

Instead, use your energy to trust. Trust that there are lessons to learn through every experience and observation, good or bad. A meaningful apology when appropriate can be an incredibly healing event but living in a continually sorry state is not where your soul wants to be. Allow your humanity to be liberated, ready to live and learn through successes and mistakes. Allow the healing balm of forgiveness to set you free.

RESISTANCE TO HEALING – PINE

But I should feel guilty! I have made mistakes and I deserve to suffer!
Making mistakes does not have to lead to suffering. Mistakes can be our gold. Trust yourself to find the lessons in the mistakes and your errors will lead to wisdom, compassion and understanding. Taking responsibility for your life is positive and helpful to yourself and others. Guilt leads nowhere and helps no one.

RED CHESTNUT

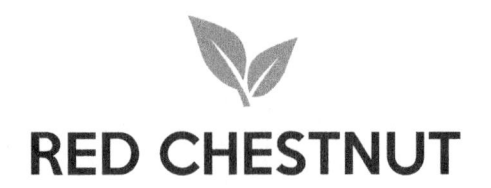

Symptoms: over-concern for the welfare of others

Positive effects: peace of mind, letting go, positivity

I am here to teach you to trust in the challenges of others. Your loved ones are here to experience human life. Within this life they will have suffering and challenges to overcome. These experiences help them develop into compassionate and wise beings. Instead of supporting them on this journey, you provide the energy of worry, panic and peril. You believe you are supporting them from a place of care, but instead you try to prevent their natural experiences, challenges and mistakes which can stunt their growth.

We ask for you, instead of focusing on all the potential pitfalls and dangers, focus on the energy you wish to surround them with. Offering a wise word of support can sometimes be helpful, but are you really just projecting fear and worry onto those around you?

When you worry for your loved ones, step back. Imagine the energy you wish for them. It could be love, support, security, gentleness, compassion, the choice is up to you. By focusing on these energies, you give them every chance of succeeding in life which is what you desired in the first place. You will become a rock of support as they feel naturally secure around the energies you are putting out, rather than the unstable, shifting sands of worry.

Caring for loved ones is a wonderful thing. By promoting peace and positivity you can be a constructive force for change in the lives of others.

RESISTANCE TO HEALING – RED CHESTNUT

But I see people in danger! If they do not watch out, they will end up in serious trouble! Take this opportunity to love yourself. This worry is within you and not in the circumstances you see before you. Send yourself the healing balm of self-love to dissolve away these concerns. The situation outside of yourself may still be challenging, but by letting go of worrying you can become a helpful, loving, supportive addition to the challenges of others.

ROCK ROSE

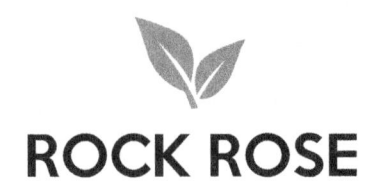

Symptoms: extreme terror, fright, panic, nightmares

Positive effects: fearlessness, security, calm

I am here to teach you about true serenity. There are times in your life when fear can become a tornado, gaining in strength, sucking up everything in its path. The fear quickens into terror and panic until you feel you can bear it no more. You are knocked off your feet, pushed and pulled as the terror and panic takes over. Calm is a memory impossible to recollect as you tumble further and further into panic.

Find the eye of the storm. In all this chaos, panic and terror there is a place of stillness, of serenity. In the very centre of it all. When you can sit quietly in the eye of your own personal storm, that is true serenity.

When a situation is terrifying, filling you with panic, search for the eye of the storm as you would look for the emergency exit sign in a fire. Everything else will be impossible until you find this stability.

You will just be thrown around getting battered and bruised until the storm passes, leaving you exhausted and surrounded by destruction. Keep focusing on this still centre. You may not find it, but do not forget it is always there. If you do find it, you have found true serenity. To be able to sit quietly within the eye of the storm, within panic and terror. To quietly observe from a place of peace as the chaos flies past.

RESISTANCE TO HEALING – ROCK ROSE

Argh! Help! I am panicking! I do not know what to do! Find the emergency exit. Get to the safe space, find the eye of the storm. Get yourself safe. Do not stop looking until you find it. Until you find safety and calm in yourself, you will only create more panic. Keep your focus on finding the eye of the storm.

ROCK WATER

Symptoms: self-denial, rigidity, strictness

Positive effects: flow, flexible, gentle

I am here to teach you to be kind to yourself. You have goals, you have values, you have ambitions. Sometimes we can become rigid, solid, like a rock, refusing to bend to anything that may come in the way of achieving our intentions.

Temptations of frivolous things such as pleasure and enjoyment will not move us from our desired outcome of goodness. We deny our nature as we see it getting in our way. But what if we can achieve our aims whilst being kinder, more gentle to ourselves?

By being rigid we resist the flow of life. Life's flows are designed to take us in certain directions, often in ways we are unaware of. By trusting in the flow our lives become rich in experiences and opportunities. When our ideas become set and we resist this flow, we limit our experiences and particularly our enjoyment. Life becomes joyless and a struggle. Opportunities are rigidly created and lack authenticity. By applying self-denial in order to achieve our goals, we deny ourselves in all areas, including the areas we are so tightly focused on. The heart grows dull, and we become lifeless.

Step back into the flow and breathe life back into your purpose. Your goals and values you so strongly believe in can still be achieved, but with much more joy and ease.

RESISTANCE TO HEALING – ROCK WATER

But I must represent this value, I must achieve this aim. At all costs. I must not be distracted by pleasure! There is a difference between avoidance and enjoyment. You fear pleasurable things and experiences are a form of avoidance. They can be, but you are avoiding life by avoiding enjoyment. Your approach is achieving the opposite of what you intend. Relax, let go and go with the flow.

SCLERANTHUS

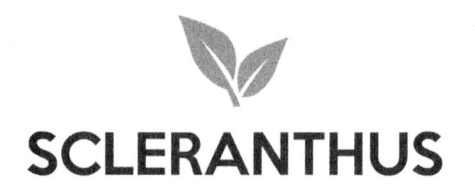

Symptoms: indecision, inability to choose

Positive effect: decisiveness, stable, balanced

I am here to teach you to allow yourself to make choices. Sometimes we have decisions to make, choices to decide. These can sometimes create such indecision within us we become paralysed in between the possibilities. We become trapped. Our only way out is through a choice; however, we fear making that choice in case it is not the perfect decision.

Slow yourself down. Give yourself a head start by getting in the best possible place for making a choice. Be still. Be quiet. Go within. If you find it hard to do this, then practise. By finding your intuition you can listen and make the best decisions from there. Or listen to your gut reaction. How does your belly feel when confronted by each choice? Or if you cannot connect to your inner feelings, by quietening your conflict, you have much more chance to use your logic to select the right choice.

Ultimately, you need to make a choice. And if it is a bad decision then you can turn it around into a lesson, deepening your wisdom. But without making that choice you remain trapped until life forces you into a situation you have not chosen which can often be very uncomfortable.

Step forward. Make a choice. Step through into the next level of experience.

RESISTANCE TO HEALING – SCLERANTHUS

But I might make a mistake! I might do it wrong! I might miss something better! Trust yourself that you will choose well just by choosing. Engage your intuition, wisdom and logic and make a choice. You have the power within you to decide what you feel is best. As long as you are choosing from a place of integrity you can't go wrong. Even if it seems to go wrong, you will gain from your choice if it comes from a place of good will.

STAR OF BETHLEHEM

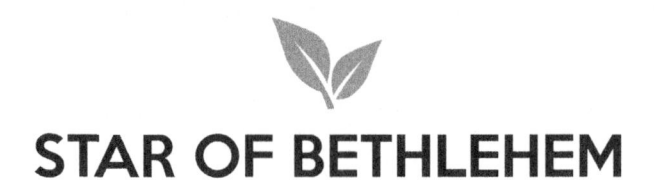

Symptoms: shock, loss, grief, trauma

Positive effects: comfort, balance, solace

I am here to teach you to be calm. Sometimes experiences can shock us to our core. This can affect us both emotionally and physically. An actual physical shock can cause trauma to the body. This is similar to how emotional shock can cause trauma. A scar might be left behind. Protective tissue that has helped us heal what needed healing most immediately. Allowing us to pick ourselves up as best we can at the time. We pick ourselves up, dust ourselves off and walk away from the shocking experience. Maybe even forgetting it. However, the scar can begin to cause its own problems. It can reopen when you least expect it, cause irritation, you might not want to look at it, nerve pain, and so on. What was initially there to help you has now become the problem.

When we do not have the ability to deal with shock in the moment, defence mechanisms are brought in, protecting us from feeling our pain. This is meant to be a temporary measure until we are ready to deal with our feelings.

I am here to help bring the calm, safe space to release. Let go. Honour the feelings. Marvel at how you protected yourself with your defence mechanisms but allow me to help soothe the flames of fear you have been keeping at bay.

RESISTANCE TO HEALING – STAR OF BETHLEHEM

I am not OK. I am not ready to deal with this. I cannot cope! We can wait until you are ready. Know that you have the ability to reclaim yourself from any situation. It might take time and that is OK. I am here to bring calm, not to retraumatise. Together we can unpick this one strand at a time. It is not always right to cut chords and let go of experiences. There is too much energy tied within them. Instead, a gentle calm unravelling is what is needed.

SWEET CHESTNUT

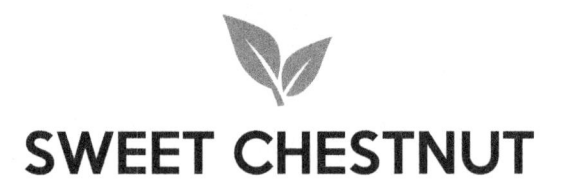

Symptoms: extreme mental anguish, no light left, despair

Positive effects: hope, support, consolation

I am here to teach you that change will always come. Sometimes life might feel like it is against us. We try everything and nothing seems to help. Exhausting all options, we are left desperate and hopeless, uncertain of how to escape. We want to find a solution, but one does not seem to come. I am here to teach you, if one thing is certain—nothing stays the same forever.

Trust. Things will change. Opportunities will come that you had not even considered. They are much easier to spot from a calm place. Can you allow yourself to just be where you are now? What do you notice in the here and now? Allow your attention to expand. The weather changes, sometimes for the worse, sometimes for the better. The temperature changes, the light, the soundscape. Now apply it to your life. All the different phases you have lived through. And there will be more!

This is a phase. Even if it is taking longer than you wish. It will pass. New opportunities will eventually appear on your horizon. Keep hope, even if you have been hoping for some time. Allow yourself to be where you are. Quieten your fears and settle into the now. Start noticing the subtle changes. One state moving into another. Moving from one polarity to the other. Always shifting, always changing.

RESISTANCE TO HEALING – SWEET CHESTNUT

But I have tried everything, and nothing seems to work. I should give up! There is nothing more I can do! Maybe you've just answered your own question there. Give up. Let go. Bring yourself back to here and now. Grasping for a different future can often hinder your progress. Come from a stiller, calmer place and allow your ever-changing future to present itself when it is ready.

VERVAIN

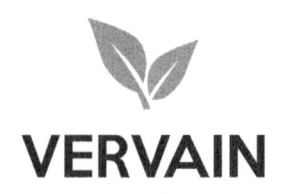

Symptoms: over-enthusiasm, fanatical

Positive effects: relaxed, tranquil

I am here to teach you how to channel your enthusiasm. Passion is a wonderful thing. It fuels life, providing a furnace to push forward ideas, concepts, actions and change. However, if this furnace is left to burn out of control it can cause destruction.

Channelled in the right way, enthusiasm can be very powerful. Like a wood burning stove, the heat is used through the relevant pipes to heat water, spaces, etc. The more efficiently the heat is contained and channelled, the more effective the power. The power is taken directly to the right places with little waste. As much energy is used positively from a piece of wood as possible.

Now put this piece of wood on an open fire. The wood can burn up rapidly; its heat disperses with little use, rising rapidly into the atmosphere. It burns up quickly into the atmosphere, and if it not monitored, the fire can spread causing untold damage.

Ideas can be the same. Enthusiasm channelled well, directly to the relevant sources, can provide so much power positively. If this is unchanneled it can be dangerous. It can push people in the opposite direction. When the fire of opinion rages so strong, it can carry people in its flames causing collective, righteous group thinking, with the potential for great destruction. It can also burn you up. If your energy is being burnt up due to overenthusiasm, your fuel is wasted and dissipates into the atmosphere.

RESISTANCE TO HEALING – VERVAIN

But I need people to see my point of view! They must change their minds! Which people? Are you wasting your energy? Is this where your fuel needs to go to be most effective? Can you channel it more effectively? Does the fire need to rage so strong, or can a steady glow provide more efficient results, and without the risk of burning the whole thing down.

VINE

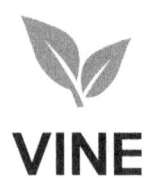

Symptoms: dominant, inflexible

Positive effects: respect, compassion

I am here to teach you to release your grip. Let it go. By trying to force things, attempting to manoeuvre people and circumstances without their consent, you play a dangerous game. Like a sergeant major you have all the commands, all the orders. You have the consequences lined up if your specified vision is not played out to perfection. You have the relevant scapegoats lined up to blame, as your vision is perfect, and the inadequacies of others cause you to fail. Maybe if you grip on tighter, they will fall into line. Or maybe you will strangle the life and love out of things.

The world is not yours to conquer. Its players are not your army. Step back.

When that inner tyrant rises, what is it trying to achieve? What are you grasping at? What are you suffocating with your grip? Have you even questioned why you are trying to make these things happen? What is under your desire to control, to enforce? Does your technique even achieve your desperate desires? If it does, it will be temporary, and the pressure of your force will cause your creations to crumble.

Release. Release. Release. Take a breath. Let go. And when you find yourself clenching, forcing, or grasping—release again. Retract your orders. At ease.

RESISTANCE TO HEALING – VINE

But if I do not force things they might not happen!

Take a breath. Listen to your motivations. Allow yourself to listen to what you are expecting. For when you try and force things you run the risk of breaking what is good around you. You run the risk of becoming a destroyer of good. Soften. Let go. Step back. Allow.

WALNUT

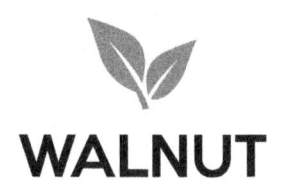

Symptoms: difficulty adapting to change and unwanted influences

Positive effects: adaptable, protected

I am here to teach you the value of transitioning from one state to another. At times in life, we are called for change. Sometimes it is our choice, sometimes circumstances, sometimes other people seemingly inflict it upon us. However it arises, this can be unsettling. Change by its very nature is unsettling. By its design.

For example, we know water can move from solid ice, to liquid water, on to vapour dispersed in the atmosphere. In order for this to happen, a change of temperature is needed, and a great deal of change happens to the molecules of water. Solid ice is warmed causing the molecules to move and vibrate until it changes form completely. Changing from a solid state to a liquid. This liquid can flow and move in a way so completely different to ice, and the same with steam.

We are like water. Circumstances change us from solid, to liquid, to gas. We are mutable as beings and have the capacity to transform and shift over and over again. This is a process of nature. Nature does not resist this change. It flows from one state to the next. As humans we often resist these transformations, sometimes to the point where we stop them from happening. The discomfort of not changing when our nature desires it becomes hard to bear. So we try to mask this discomfort in various ways, which can lead to multiple problems. Eventually we have to change, but this process becomes much harder than if we had just allowed it in the first place. Let yourself melt, let yourself evaporate, let yourself solidify.

RESISTANCE TO HEALING – WALNUT

But I do not want to change! It is too difficult. There are too many reasons to stay the same! Can you imagine water reaching melting point and trying to stay solid ice? When its nature wanted to be fluid, liquid and expressive. Trying to stay solid, stationary and hard? The amount of effort it takes to maintain a form which is ready to transition into something else will only lead to more problems, more discomfort, more unnecessary effort. Change is nature.

WATER VIOLET

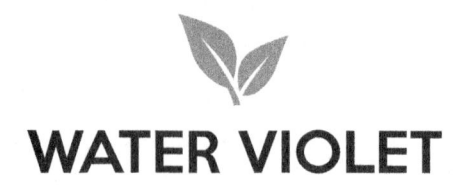

Symptoms: proud, aloof, isolation

Positive effects: connection, communication, warmth

I am here to teach you how to connect. Isolation can sometimes become a place of comfort. To be by oneself is indeed a sanctuary. It is a gift to enjoy. But it can lead to separation from others. Separation to a degree where other people become unnecessary in your life. You develop a cold reserve, as you know you can cope by yourself. You can manage just fine. But by having this self-reliance you can begin to move through life missing out.

We are here to be part of the game of life. To experience, to be in relation with other beings. Other people. We need connections or we miss out on one of the most valuable aspects of being human. Relationships. To relate to others is where we find most of our growth, most of our learning, most of our comfort, and indeed, most of our joy. However, it is also difficult to live alongside others because there is such rich learning within these relationships.

Whereas some people fear being alone, some become resistant to company. I am here to teach you how connection is life. It does not get in the way of life. That thing you are trying to avoid so you can carry on fine, just as you are, is the very thing your soul wants to experience.

RESISTANCE TO HEALING – WATER VIOLET

But I am fine on my own. I can look after myself. I do not need anyone else. But is this enough? Would life not be so much more if you shared some of it with others? Would the depth of your experience not widen with new perspectives, new connections? And would others not miss out on the wonder that is you? Connection is more valuable than most things. It is why we are here. Enjoy it as much as you enjoy solitude!

WHITE CHESTNUT

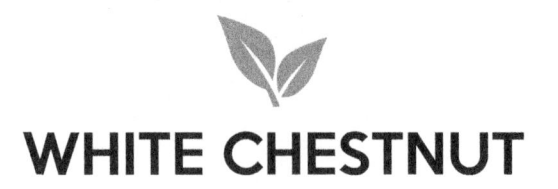

Symptoms: obsessive thoughts, mental arguments

Positive effects: tranquil, quiet, still

I am here to show you peace. I am here to show you the efficiency of a quiet mind.

Your thoughts rattle around your mind over and over, round and round. No beginning and no end. Chasing their tail, running down dead ends, considering everything, concluding nothing. This is the emotional equivalent of running a marathon, but there is no medal at the end. Only mental exhaustion, lack of sleep and wasted time.

See these restless, repetitive thoughts like an overexcited toddler. Trying to explore everything in a disjointed, hyperactive way. It seems fun at the time, but as the ferocity of exploration ramps up, it is harder to think straight, nothing becomes satisfying, and overtired tears of confusion come.

Stop winding yourself up. Watch your mind and calm it down. This may not be easy but it is a practice. A practice of peace. Give yourself a chance of peace by noticing when your mind toddles off. If left unwatched, it can wander into confusing areas, leading to distraction and distress. Take yourself by the hand and lead yourself back to peace. Over and over and over again.

Eventually, you will realise that a peaceful mind is the space where the most valuable thoughts can seed themselves. These thoughts are quiet thoughts. They cannot be heard within the clutter, amongst the rampaging of unruly toddlers. Their whispers are heard in peace.

RESISTANCE TO HEALING – WHITE CHESTNUT

But I just cannot stop the thoughts! I try but they keep going round and round! Then do not try and stop them. Gently practise reminding yourself of a peaceful mind. Keep leading yourself towards peace. Rather than chastising the chattering mind, turn in the direction of peace. There is a time when peace will become the familiar landscape of your mind. Until then, keep practising leading your mind back to peace.

WILD OAT

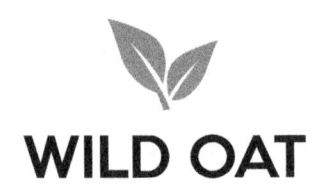

Symptoms: uncertainty over direction in life

Positive effects: purpose, direction, satisfied

I am here to show you the meaning of purpose. Purpose can mean different things to different people. Purpose can be found in the simplest things in life. Great feelings of purpose can be found whilst folding the laundry, whilst booking train tickets, whilst doing the washing up. If you feel like you have not found your purpose in life, if you feel you are searching for that special thing that sets your heart on fire, find the purpose in what's in front of you now.

When you start to live with purpose, life becomes more meaningful. Those moment when you are living in autopilot have the potential to become rich with significance and value.

Some people know their destiny, whether that be a nurse, a teacher, a train driver, a parent, or anything else. This is wonderful. However, if this purpose is not clear to you, it does not mean your life has no meaning. Life itself is your purpose. You yourself are your purpose. Rather than searching for your purpose, feel purposeful. Bring your full self into each moment. When you have a menial task to do, fill it with significance, meaning and purpose. Allow yourself to give yourself fully to the task at hand, drop into it and witness your role in the great tapestry of life.

As you practise life with purpose it will fill your experience more and more. You will notice it all around. Opportunities will become laden with purpose. Gradually you will come to see you are living the life you are meant to live.

RESISTANCE TO HEALING – WILD OAT

But I am wasting my life! I cannot find what I am meant to do!
By searching with a sense of dissatisfaction, you will only find dissatisfaction. Open your eyes to purpose, to meaning, and you will discover the void you have known slowly begins to fill. Your life will become worthwhile, and you will discover your role in the world.

WILD ROSE

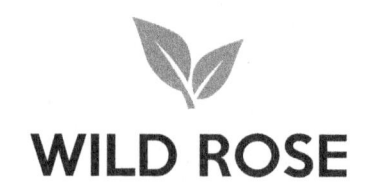

Symptoms: drifting, resignation, apathy

Positive effect: enthusiasm, engaged, ambition

I am here to teach you to rise up. To becoming the full version of yourself. Sometimes in life it is easy to become happy with your lot. It could be better, it could be worse. Best not to rock the boat.

By drifting through life, doing just enough, no more, no less, we become numb to the wonder of life. We become numb to the richness of what we can be. The potential struggle, and hard work involved in becoming all we could be, is so far from feeling settled in our comfort zone.

Apathy is a form of death. Our light gradually dims as parts of us are turned off. Our youthful dreams are faded, and we tread water through life, taking the easy route where we can. We become numb. We are resigned to our mediocre life anticipating nothing special.

Wake up! Wake up now! You are slumbering in what could be the most wonderful life. You could be the hero in this story, but instead you are part of the supporting cast. Blending into the background, making little impact on the plot.

You came here to live! You are ready to come fully alive. Wake up! The time is now! Appreciate who you are and what you came here to do.

Drifting downstream whilst fully awake is the key. Letting life flow with your eyes wide open. Not drifting half asleep, half alive, numb with your eyes shut. Wake up!

RESISTANCE TO HEALING – WILD ROSE

But I want an easy life. I do not want to push myself. Let me take it easy! You are confusing being relaxed and in flow with avoidance and apathy. You are half alive. There is so much to live, and you are not living it. This is your wake-up call. The time is now. Wake up, wake up, wake up!

WILLOW

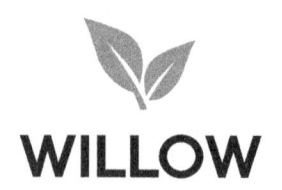

Symptoms: self-pity, resentment

Positive effects: forgiveness, responsibility, positivity

I am here to teach you to see the good around you. To see the support you have. To see the magnificence of the resources surrounding you.

Sometimes in life it is easy to become disheartened. You notice how life seems to be working against you. You are a victim of your circumstances, and you know it. The way you move through life is with regret and resentment over the cards you have been dealt. You glance over at other people's hands of cards and wonder why they got dealt all the aces. It is not fair!

Well shuffle the deck. Know that your luck can change with each deal of the cards. Let go of your past misfortune and look forward with hope. Next time you might be the one with the strong hand. Until then, celebrate those who are winning at life. Remember that their success does not take away from yours. Rather than seeing yourself as the victim of life, see those around you giving glimpses of what your potential could be, rather than them highlighting your misfortune.

Life can be difficult, painful and traumatic. But it can change. By living in resentment, you are tied into misfortune and injustice. It is tied into your experience.

Foster hope into your life. Expect good things alongside the misfortune. Life is a spectrum of experience. Turn around and expect a change in fortune.

RESISTANCE TO HEALING – WILLOW

But life's not fair. Why do I get such a tough time? Why do others have it so easy? Why can't you celebrate the people who demonstrate the good, enjoyable aspects of life, instead of resenting them? Give thanks for other people's successes. And give thanks for your own, no matter how small. Do you have a roof over your head? You do? Wonderful! How lucky you are! Do you have health in some areas of your body? You do? That's great! Keep building gratitude for yourself and for others. Let the good parts in too.

ACKNOWLEDGEMENTS

I wish to thank firstly, the Bach Flower Remedies, who are the true authors of this book. I feel honoured to assist them in the creation of bringing their words to the page.

To Dr Bach and the legacy he left, which is still inspiring myself and so many others. In gratitude for the healing and transformation his remedies have provided.

I'm forever grateful to my guides, teachers and fellow essence producers, who have taught me so much and continue to do so, and have helped light the way to my finding this wonderous path I now walk.

To all those that have contributed to my remembering that I am part of nature and how to enter that magical space of connection and communication.

To Michelle, for your skills in helping me get this book off my computer and into the world.

Thanks to Matthew for your reading and reflecting. I appreciate your love, support, honesty and integrity, both with this book and in life.

Thanks to my parents for their support in so many ways.

And finally, thanks to nature and all she provides.

ABOUT THE AUTHOR

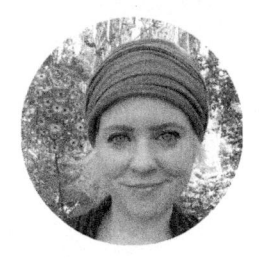

Helen Scott is an Advanced Flower and Vibrational Essence Practitioner, member of the BFVEA (British Flower and Vibrational Essence Association), and BAFEP (British Association of Flower Essence Producers). She is the founder of Super Nature, and the producer of the Super Nature Vibrational Essences.

Having used essences throughout her life, and in her work as a holistic practitioner, Helen is passionate about sharing the wonders of flower and vibrational essences and the gentle, healing power of nature.

She currently spends her time between her home in Manchester and roaming around the British Isles creating essences, deepening her relationship to nature and the wisdom and joy it holds.

Her work is based at Studio Super Nature, a portal to nature in a Victorian mill in the industrial heartland of Manchester, in the north of England.

Discover more about her work, offerings, and the Super Nature Essences at: **studiosupernature.com**

Printed in Great Britain
by Amazon